Paleo Diet Easy to Use Guide for Beginners

The Benefit of Making Paleo Diet as a Lifestyle

By

Eoghan Brady

Table of Contents

CHAPTER 1

Introduction

1.1 Understanding the Paleo Diet

The Paleo Diet, short for the Paleolithic Diet, is a dietary approach that seeks to mimic the eating patterns of our ancient ancestors from the Paleolithic era, which spanned from about 2.5 million to 10,000 years ago. This diet is rooted in the belief that our bodies are best adapted to the types of foods our hunter-gatherer ancestors consumed, long before the advent of agriculture and modern food processing.

At its core, the Paleo Diet emphasizes the consumption of whole, unprocessed foods that would have been available to our ancestors. This includes lean meats, fish, poultry, fruits, vegetables, nuts, and seeds while excluding grains, dairy products, legumes, refined sugars, and processed foods.

The foundational principle behind the Paleo Diet is that it aligns with our evolutionary biology. Proponents argue that our genetic makeup has changed very little since the Paleolithic era, and as such, our bodies are still best suited to the diet of that time. By consuming foods that our bodies are inherently adapted to, we can potentially improve our overall health and well-being.

1.2 Benefits of the Paleo Diet

The Paleo Diet has gained popularity due to several potential health benefits it claims to offer:

a. Weight Management: One of the primary benefits associated with the Paleo Diet is its potential to aid in weight management. The diet is naturally low in processed foods, added sugars, and refined carbohydrates, which can contribute to weight loss or maintenance.

b. Improved Blood Sugar Control: Some individuals find that the Paleo Diet can help stabilize blood sugar levels, which is beneficial for those with diabetes or those at risk of developing the condition.

c. Enhanced Nutrient Intake: The emphasis on whole foods means that the Paleo Diet can be rich in essential nutrients, including vitamins, minerals, and antioxidants, which are vital for overall health.

d. Better Digestive Health: By eliminating grains and legumes, which contain compounds that can be hard to digest for some people, the Paleo Diet may improve digestive health and reduce digestive discomfort.

e. Increased Protein Intake: The diet typically encourages higher protein intake, which can aid in muscle maintenance and promote a feeling of fullness.

f. Reduction in Inflammation: The avoidance of processed and inflammatory foods may lead to reduced inflammation in the body, potentially benefiting individuals with inflammatory conditions.

g. Enhanced Energy Levels: Some individuals report increased energy levels and improved overall well-being when following the Paleo Diet.

1.3 Is the Paleo Diet Right for You?

While the Paleo Diet has gained a dedicated following and offers several potential health benefits, it's essential to consider whether it's the right dietary choice for you. Here are some factors to contemplate:

a. Personal Health Goals: Assess your health and wellness objectives. If you're looking to lose weight, manage blood sugar, or improve digestive health, the Paleo Diet might align with your goals.

b. Dietary Preferences: Consider your dietary preferences and restrictions. If you have a strong preference for whole, unprocessed foods and are not attached to grains, dairy, or legumes, the Paleo Diet may be easier to adopt.

c. Lifestyle and Convenience: Evaluate how well the diet fits into your lifestyle. The Paleo Diet can require more meal preparation and planning than some other dietary patterns.

d. Individual Health Needs: Consult with a healthcare professional, especially if you have specific health conditions or dietary concerns. They can provide personalized guidance on whether the Paleo Diet is suitable for you.

e. Long-Term Sustainability: Think about whether you can see yourself maintaining this way of eating over the long term. Sustainable dietary changes are more likely to yield lasting benefits.

The Paleo Diet is a dietary approach rooted in evolutionary principles that can offer various health benefits. However, whether it's the right choice for you depends on your individual health goals, dietary preferences, and lifestyle. Consulting with a healthcare professional can help you make an informed decision about whether to adopt the Paleo Diet as part of your overall health and wellness plan.

CHAPTER 2

The Basics of the Paleo Diet

2.1 What Is Allowed on the Paleo Diet?

The Paleo Diet focuses on whole, unprocessed foods that our ancestors from the Paleolithic era would have consumed. Here's a breakdown of what is typically allowed on the Paleo Diet:

a. Lean Meats: This includes poultry, such as chicken and turkey, as well as lean cuts of beef, pork, and lamb. Grass-fed and pasture-raised meats are often preferred for their healthier fat profile.

b. Fish and Seafood: Fatty fish like salmon, mackerel, and sardines are rich in omega-3 fatty acids and are staples of the Paleo Diet. Shellfish like shrimp and crab are also included.

c. Fruits: A variety of fresh fruits are encouraged, including berries, apples, oranges, and bananas. These provide natural sweetness and essential vitamins and minerals.

d. Vegetables: Non-starchy vegetables are a cornerstone of the diet. Options like broccoli, spinach, kale, carrots, and cauliflower are commonly consumed.

e. Nuts and Seeds: Almonds, walnuts, cashews, and seeds like chia, flax, and pumpkin seeds are allowed. They offer healthy fats and protein.

f. Healthy Fats and Oils: Avocado, olive oil, coconut oil, and ghee (clarified butter) are preferred sources of fats. These fats are considered more natural and less processed than many vegetable oils.

g. Eggs: Eggs are a rich source of protein and are typically included in the Paleo Diet.

h. Herbs and Spices: A wide range of herbs and spices can be used for flavoring without the need for processed condiments.

i. Natural Sweeteners (in moderation): Occasional use of honey and maple syrup is permitted, but it's essential to use them sparingly due to their sugar content.

j. Beverages: Water is the primary beverage on the Paleo Diet. Herbal teas, and some advocates allow for moderate consumption of black coffee, are generally acceptable.

2.2 What to Avoid on the Paleo Diet

The Paleo Diet restricts or eliminates certain food groups that were not part of our ancestors' diets:

a. Grains: All grains, including wheat, rice, corn, and oats, are excluded. This means no bread, pasta, or cereal.

b. Dairy: Dairy products, including milk, cheese, and yogurt, are typically avoided. Some Paleo followers make exceptions for small amounts of high-fat dairy like butter or ghee.

c. Legumes: Beans, lentils, peanuts, and other legumes are not allowed due to their lectin and phytate content, which can be hard to digest for some people.

d. Processed Foods: Highly processed foods, such as sugary snacks, sodas, and most packaged foods, are off-limits.

e. Refined Sugars: Foods and beverages high in refined sugars, like candies, pastries, and sugary drinks, are to be avoided.

f. Vegetable Oils: Most vegetable oils, such as soybean, corn, and canola oil, are excluded due to their high omega-6 fatty acid content.

g. Artificial Additives: Artificial sweeteners, preservatives, and flavor enhancers are not part of the Paleo Diet.

2.3 The Philosophy Behind Paleo

The philosophy behind the Paleo Diet is rooted in the belief that our bodies are best adapted to the foods our pre-agricultural ancestors consumed during the Paleolithic era. Proponents argue that our genetic makeup has changed very little since that time, and our modern health problems are partly attributed to the consumption of processed and unnatural foods that emerged with the advent of agriculture and industrialization.

The key principles of the Paleo philosophy include:

a. Whole, Unprocessed Foods: Emphasizing natural, unprocessed foods that are nutrient-dense and free from artificial additives.

b. Nutrient Density: Focusing on foods rich in essential nutrients, such as vitamins, minerals, and antioxidants, to support overall health.

c. Elimination of Modern Culprits: Avoiding foods that are thought to contribute to modern health issues, such as grains, dairy, and processed sugars.

d. Embracing Healthy Fats: Encouraging the consumption of healthy fats like those found in avocados, nuts, and fatty fish.

e. Personalization: Acknowledging that individual tolerance to certain foods can vary, so the diet can be adapted to suit individual needs.

The Paleo Diet seeks to provide a framework for a more natural and healthful way of eating, based on the presumed dietary patterns of our distant ancestors. However, it's important to note that while the diet has its proponents, it also has its critics who argue that it oversimplifies the complexities of modern nutrition and that the historical accuracy of the diet's assumptions is debated. As with any diet, it's crucial to consider your individual health goals, preferences, and consult with a healthcare professional before making significant dietary changes.

CHAPTER 3

Getting Started with the Paleo Diet

3.1 Preparing Your Kitchen

Before diving into the Paleo Diet, it's essential to prepare your kitchen to make the transition smoother and set yourself up for success. Here's how you can get started:

a. Clean Out Your Pantry: Begin by removing non-Paleo items from your pantry, refrigerator, and freezer. This includes grains, legumes, dairy products, and processed foods. Donate or discard items you won't be using.

b. Stock Up on Paleo Staples:
Replace eliminated items with Paleo-friendly alternatives. Make sure you have a variety of lean meats, fish, eggs, fresh vegetables, fruits, nuts, and seeds on hand.

c. Invest in Kitchen Tools: Equip your kitchen with essential tools for preparing Paleo meals, such as a good chef's knife, cutting boards, a blender or food processor, and a range of pots and pans for cooking different foods.

d. Meal Prep Containers: Consider purchasing meal prep containers to make it easier to store and portion your Paleo meals.

e. Organize Your Kitchen: Arrange your kitchen so that Paleo-friendly foods are easily accessible. Keep fresh fruits and vegetables at eye level in the refrigerator, and store nuts and seeds in clear containers for quick and healthy snacks.

f. Learn New Cooking Techniques: Familiarize yourself with cooking methods that align with the Paleo Diet, such as grilling, roasting, stir-frying, and baking. These techniques will help you prepare delicious and nutritious meals.

3.2 Planning Your Meals

Effective meal planning is key to maintaining a successful Paleo Diet. Here's a guide to help you plan your Paleo meals:

a. Create a Weekly Meal Plan: Sit down and plan your meals for the week. This includes breakfast, lunch, dinner, and any snacks. Having a plan reduces the temptation to resort to non-Paleo foods when you're hungry and in a hurry.

b. Balance Your Macronutrients: Ensure that your meals are well-balanced with lean protein, healthy fats, and a variety of colorful vegetables. Include some fruits, nuts, and seeds for added nutrients and flavor.

c. Experiment with Recipes: There are numerous Paleo recipes available in cookbooks and online. Experiment with different recipes to keep your meals interesting and flavorful. Don't be afraid to get creative in the kitchen.

d. Batch Cooking: Consider batch cooking on weekends or your days off. Prepare larger quantities of Paleo dishes that can be portioned and frozen for later use. This can save you time during busy weekdays.

e. Pre-Pack Snacks: Prepare Paleo-friendly snacks in advance, such as carrot sticks with almond butter, for quick and healthy munching.

f. Listen to Your Body: Pay attention to your body's hunger and fullness cues. The Paleo Diet emphasizes eating whole, nutrient-dense foods, but it's also important to eat in a way that suits your individual needs and lifestyle.

3.3 Grocery Shopping for Paleo-Friendly Foods

Navigating the grocery store for Paleo-friendly foods can be straightforward with a bit of planning. Here's how to approach your grocery shopping:

a. Make a Shopping List: Before heading to the store, make a list of the items you need based on your meal plan. Stick to your list to avoid impulse purchases.

b. Shop the Perimeter: In most grocery stores, the perimeter is where you'll find fresh produce, meats, and seafood. These sections will be your primary focus.

c. Choose Quality Meats: opt for grass-fed or pasture-raised meats whenever possible. They tend to have a better nutrient profile than conventionally raised animals.

d. Load Up on Vegetables: Buy a variety of colorful vegetables to ensure a wide range of nutrients in your diet. Fresh or frozen options are both suitable.

e. Select Seasonal Fruits: Choose seasonal fruits for freshness and affordability.

f. Explore the Bulk Aisle: The bulk aisle often has nuts, seeds, and dried fruits. You can buy these items in the quantities you need.

g. Read Labels Carefully: When buying packaged foods, read labels to ensure they meet Paleo guidelines. Look for minimal ingredients and avoid products with additives or preservatives.

h. Be Mindful of Oils: Check your cooking oils to make sure they align with the Paleo Diet. Olive oil, coconut oil, and avocado oil are good choices.

i. Plan for Snacks: Have Paleo-friendly snacks like nuts, fruit, or jerky on hand to satisfy cravings.

j. Avoid Impulse Buys: Stay disciplined and avoid buying non-Paleo items, especially when you encounter tempting displays or promotions.

k. Stay Hydrated: Remember to pick up plenty of water or herbal teas to stay well-hydrated.

Preparing your kitchen, planning your meals, and shopping strategically, you can make the transition to the Paleo Diet more manageable and enjoyable. With practice, you'll become adept at selecting and preparing delicious, Paleo-friendly dishes that support your health and well-being.

CHAPTER 4

Building Balanced Paleo Meals

Building balanced Paleo meals is essential to ensure you're getting the right mix of nutrients for optimal health and well-being. Here's a guide on how to create well-rounded Paleo dishes:

4.1 Incorporating Lean Proteins

Protein is a crucial component of the Paleo Diet, as it helps with muscle maintenance, satiety, and overall health. Here's how to incorporate lean proteins into your meals:

a. Lean Meats: Include lean cuts of beef, poultry (chicken, turkey), and pork in your diet. Opt for grass-fed or pasture-raised meats when possible, as they tend to have a better nutrient profile.

b. Fatty Fish: Enjoy fatty fish like salmon, mackerel, and sardines for their omega-3 fatty acids. These are essential for heart and brain health.

c. Eggs: Eggs are an excellent source of protein and can be prepared in various ways, such as scrambled, poached, or boiled.

d. Seafood: Incorporate a variety of seafood like shrimp, crab, and scallops for lean protein and essential minerals.

e. Poultry: Skinless chicken and turkey breasts are lean protein options. Consider grilling, baking, or roasting them for a healthy meal.

f. Game Meats: If available and appealing to you, consider game meats like bison, venison, or rabbit for a change of taste and additional nutrients.

4.2 Choosing Nutrient-Rich Vegetables

Vegetables are a cornerstone of the Paleo Diet, providing essential vitamins, minerals, and fiber. Here's how to choose nutrient-rich vegetables:

a. Go Colorful: Aim for a variety of colorful vegetables, as different colors often indicate different nutrients. Include leafy greens, carrots, bell peppers, broccoli, and cauliflower.

b. Eat Seasonally: Seasonal vegetables tend to be fresher, tastier, and more affordable. Visit local farmers' markets for a selection of seasonal produce.

c. Experiment with Cooking Methods: Try different cooking methods like roasting, steaming, or sautéing to find your favorite way to prepare vegetables.

d. Consider Starchy Vegetables in Moderation: While starchy vegetables like sweet potatoes and butternut squash are allowed on the Paleo Diet, consume them in moderation due to their higher carbohydrate content.

e. Organic Options: If possible, choose organic vegetables to reduce exposure to pesticides and support sustainable farming practices.

4.3 Healthy Fats and Oils

Healthy fats and oils are an integral part of the Paleo Diet. They provide essential fatty acids and enhance the flavor of your meals. Here's how to incorporate them:

a. Avocado: Avocado is a versatile and nutritious source of healthy fats. Add sliced avocado to salads or mash it for guacamole.

b. Olive Oil: Extra virgin olive oil is an excellent choice for salad dressings and low-heat cooking.

c. Coconut Oil: Use coconut oil for medium-heat cooking and baking. It adds a pleasant tropical flavor to dishes.

d. Nuts and Seeds: Almonds, walnuts, chia seeds, and flaxseeds are rich in healthy fats. Add them to salads, yogurt, or enjoy them as a snack.

e. Nut Butters: Natural nut butters (without added sugar or hydrogenated oils) can be used as spreads or in smoothies.

f. Ghee: Clarified butter (ghee) is suitable for cooking at higher temperatures and has a rich, buttery flavor.

4.4 Including Fruits and Nuts

Fruits and nuts add natural sweetness, flavor, and texture to your Paleo meals. Here's how to include them:

a. Fresh Fruits: Consume a variety of fresh fruits such as berries, apples, oranges, and bananas. Enjoy them as snacks, in smoothies, or as a side dish.

b. Dried Fruits (in moderation): Dried fruits can be higher in sugar and calories, so consume them in moderation. Look for options without added sugars or preservatives.

c. Nuts and Seeds: Include almonds, walnuts, cashews, and seeds like chia, flax, and pumpkin seeds in your diet for healthy fats and protein. They make great additions to salads and are perfect for snacking.

d. Nut Butter: Spread natural nut butter on fruit slices or use it as a dip for vegetables.

e. Fruity Desserts: When you're craving something sweet, consider fruit salads, baked apples, or a medley of berries topped with a drizzle of honey.

Incorporating lean proteins, nutrient-rich vegetables, healthy fats and oils, fruits, and nuts into your Paleo meals, you can create balanced and satisfying dishes that support your nutritional needs and align with the principles of the Paleo Diet. Remember to personalize your meals to suit your taste preferences and dietary goals.

CHAPTER 5

Sample Paleo Meal Plans

Creating a sample Paleo meal plan can be a helpful way to get started on the Paleo Diet. Here's a one-week meal plan for beginners, followed by tips on adjusting meal plans to your specific needs.

5.1 One-Week Meal Plan for Beginners

Day 1:

Breakfast: Scrambled eggs with spinach and tomatoes, topped with avocado slices. **Lunch:** Grilled chicken breast salad with mixed greens, cherry tomatoes, cucumber, and a balsamic vinaigrette dressing. **Snack:** Carrot and celery sticks with almond butter. **Dinner:** Baked salmon with roasted asparagus and a side of mashed sweet potatoes.

Day 2:

Breakfast: A smoothie with spinach, banana, almond milk, and a scoop of protein powder. **Lunch:** Turkey and avocado lettuce wraps with a side of sliced bell peppers. **Snack:** Mixed berries and a handful of raw nuts. **Dinner:** Stir-fried shrimp with broccoli, bell peppers, and cauliflower rice.

Day 3:

Breakfast: Omelet with mushrooms, onions, and bell peppers. **Lunch:** Leftover stir-fried shrimp from Day 2.

Snack: Sliced apple with almond butter. **Dinner:** Grilled flank steak with sautéed kale and garlic.

Day 4:

Breakfast: Greek yogurt topped with berries and chopped nuts (if dairy is tolerated). **Lunch:** Tuna salad with mixed greens, olives, and a lemon vinaigrette dressing. **Snack:** Cherry tomatoes with guacamole. **Dinner:** Baked chicken thighs with roasted Brussels sprouts and a side of butternut squash soup.

Day 5:

Breakfast: Scrambled eggs with diced ham and sautéed bell peppers. **Lunch:** Spinach and kale salad with grilled shrimp, cherry tomatoes, and a homemade avocado dressing. **Snack:** Sliced cucumbers with tzatziki sauce. **Dinner:** Baked cod with steamed broccoli and a side of cauliflower mash.

Day 6:

Breakfast: Coconut milk chia pudding with sliced strawberries and a drizzle of honey. **Lunch:** Leftover cod and cauliflower mash from Day 5. **Snack:** Mixed nuts and dried fruits (in moderation). **Dinner:** Beef and vegetable stir-fry with a coconut aminos sauce.

Day 7:

Breakfast: Baked avocado and eggs with a sprinkle of bacon bits. **Lunch:** Grilled chicken salad with mixed greens, roasted red peppers, and a paleo-friendly ranch dressing. **Snack:** Sliced pear with a small serving of almond butter. **Dinner:** Pork tenderloin with sautéed spinach and mashed turnips.

5.2 Adjusting Meal Plans to Your Needs

Adjusting a Paleo meal plan to your specific needs involves considering factors such as dietary restrictions, calorie requirements, and taste preferences. Here are some tips:

a. Dietary Restrictions: If you have dietary restrictions or allergies (e.g., nut allergies or lactose intolerance), be sure to choose substitutes that align with your needs. For instance, replace almond butter with sunflower seed butter if you have nut allergies.

b. Calorie Requirements: Adjust portion sizes and the number of snacks to meet your daily calorie needs. If you're aiming for weight loss, you might need to reduce portion sizes, but be mindful not to excessively restrict calories.

c. Taste Preferences: Customize the meal plan to your taste preferences. If you dislike certain vegetables, swap them for others you enjoy. Experiment with seasonings and spices to add variety to your meals.

d. Meal Timing: Adapt meal timing to your schedule. If you prefer larger breakfasts and lighter dinners or need more snacks throughout the day, adjust accordingly.

e. Food Availability: Choose foods that are readily available in your region to ensure freshness and affordability.

f. Supplements: Consider adding supplements like vitamin D or omega-3 fatty acids if you're concerned about meeting specific nutrient needs.

g. Social and Dining Out: Plan for social occasions and dining out by making Paleo-friendly choices when possible. Look for restaurants that offer Paleo-friendly options or eat a balanced meal before going out to reduce temptations.

That meal planning is flexible, and it's essential to tailor it to your individual needs and goals. As you become more familiar with the Paleo Diet and how your body responds to it, you can further refine your meal plans to optimize your health and well-being.

CHAPTER 6
Cooking and Food Preparation

Cooking and food preparation are integral aspects of the Paleo Diet. This section covers Paleo-friendly cooking techniques, natural flavoring options, and provides some quick and easy Paleo recipes.

6.1 Paleo-Friendly Cooking Techniques

The Paleo Diet emphasizes whole, unprocessed foods, and certain cooking techniques work particularly well to prepare these foods:

a. Grilling: Grilling is a fantastic way to cook lean meats, poultry, and vegetables. It imparts a smoky flavor and allows excess fat to drip away.

b. Roasting: Roasting vegetables and meats in the oven brings out their natural sweetness and flavors. Coat vegetables in olive oil and your choice of herbs and spices for added taste.

c. Sautéing: Sautéing in olive oil or coconut oil is a quick way to cook vegetables, meats, or seafood while preserving their texture and flavor.

d. Steaming: Steaming vegetables is a gentle method that retains their nutrients and vibrant colors. It's perfect for broccoli, cauliflower, and leafy greens.

e. Stir-Frying: Stir-frying with coconut aminos or other Paleo-friendly sauces is a great way to create flavorful, Asian-inspired dishes with lots of vegetables and lean protein.

f. Baking: Baking is versatile for preparing dishes like casseroles, frittatas, and roasted chicken. Use almond meal or coconut flour as a breadcrumb substitute for coating meats or vegetables.

g. Slow Cooking: Slow cookers are perfect for making Paleo-friendly stews, soups, and braised dishes. The long cooking time tenderizes meats and infuses flavors.

h. Raw Food: Incorporate raw foods like salads and fresh fruit into your diet for their natural flavors and nutrient content.

6.2 Flavoring Your Dishes Naturally

Paleo cooking doesn't rely on processed sauces and seasonings. Instead, enhance your dishes with these natural flavoring options:

a. Fresh Herbs: Use fresh herbs like basil, cilantro, parsley, and rosemary to add freshness and depth to your dishes.

b. Garlic and Onions: These aromatic ingredients provide savory flavor to many Paleo recipes.

c. Citrus: Lemon and lime juice or zest can brighten up a dish with a burst of acidity.

d. Vinegar: Balsamic, apple cider, or red wine vinegar can be used to create tangy dressings and marinades.

e. Spices: Experiment with Paleo-friendly spices such as cumin, paprika, turmeric, and chili powder for depth of flavor.

f. Coconut Aminos: This soy sauce alternative adds a salty and slightly sweet flavor to stir-fries and marinades.

g. Mustard: Dijon or whole-grain mustard can be used as a condiment or to create tangy sauces.

h. Nutritional Yeast: For a cheesy flavor, consider nutritional yeast, which is often used as a dairy-free alternative.

i. Homemade Sauces: Create your own Paleo-friendly sauces, like tomato sauce using fresh tomatoes and herbs or a creamy avocado-based dressing.

6.3 Quick and Easy Paleo Recipes

Here are three quick and easy Paleo recipes to get you started:

1. Grilled Lemon Herb Chicken:

- Ingredients:

  - 4 boneless, skinless chicken breasts

  - Juice of 1 lemon

  - Fresh herbs (e.g., rosemary, thyme, basil)

  - Salt and pepper to taste

- Instructions:

  - Marinate chicken in lemon juice, herbs, salt, and pepper for 15-30 minutes.

- Preheat grill to medium-high heat.

- Grill chicken for 6-8 minutes per side or until fully cooked.

2. Sautéed Garlic Spinach:

- Ingredients:

  - 1 bunch of fresh spinach

  - 2 cloves garlic, minced

  - 1 tablespoon olive oil

  - Salt and pepper to taste

- Instructions:

  - Heat olive oil in a pan over medium heat.

  - Add minced garlic and sauté for 1-2 minutes.

  - Add spinach and cook until wilted.

- Season with salt and pepper.

3. Baked Salmon with Roasted Vegetables:

- Ingredients:

  - 4 salmon fillets

  - Assorted vegetables (e.g., carrots, broccoli, bell peppers)

  - Olive oil

  - Lemon zest

  - Fresh dill

  - Salt and pepper to taste

- Instructions:

  - Preheat the oven to 375°F (190°C).

  - Toss vegetables with olive oil, lemon zest, dill, salt, and pepper.

- Place salmon fillets on a baking sheet and surround them with the vegetables.

- Bake for 15-20 minutes or until the salmon flakes easily with a fork.

These recipes showcase the simplicity and deliciousness of Paleo cooking. Feel free to modify them to suit your taste preferences and explore other Paleo-friendly ingredients and flavor combinations to create your own unique dishes.

CHAPTER 7

Navigating Social Situations and Challenges

Maintaining a Paleo lifestyle in social situations and overcoming common challenges can be challenging but is entirely manageable with some strategies and preparation. Here are some tips for navigating social situations and common challenges on the Paleo Diet:

7.1 Eating Paleo at Restaurants

Eating at restaurants while following the Paleo Diet can be enjoyable and stress-free with a few simple steps:

a. Research the Menu: Before going to a restaurant, check out their menu online if available. Look for dishes that naturally align with Paleo principles, such as salads, grilled meats, and seafood.

b. Call Ahead: If you have specific dietary needs, consider calling the restaurant in advance to inquire about Paleo-friendly options or request modifications to existing dishes.

c. Custom Orders: Don't hesitate to customize your order. Ask for substitutions like extra vegetables instead of grains or a salad instead of fries.

d. Skip the Bread: Politely decline bread or other non-Paleo items that may be offered as an appetizer.

e. Sauce on the Side: Request sauces and dressings on the side, so you can control the amount you use.

f. Be Clear About Allergies: If you have food allergies or intolerances, communicate them clearly to the server to avoid any potential issues.

g. Stay Mindful of Portions: Restaurant portions can be large. Consider sharing a dish with someone or taking leftovers home.

7.2 Managing Paleo at Social Gatherings

Social gatherings often involve foods that may not align with the Paleo Diet, but you can still enjoy them while staying true to your eating principles:

a. Bring Your Own Dish: If it's appropriate, offer to bring a Paleo-friendly dish to share. This ensures you have something to eat and introduces others to Paleo-friendly options.

b. Communicate with the Host: If you're comfortable doing so, talk to the host about your dietary preferences and ask if they can accommodate your needs or provide information about the planned menu.

c. Eat Beforehand: If you're unsure about the available food options, eat a small Paleo-friendly meal or snack before the event to curb your appetite.

d. Focus on the Social Aspect: Instead of making food the central focus of social gatherings, engage in conversations and enjoy the company of friends and family.

e. Be Respectful: Be polite and gracious if you choose not to eat certain foods. People may have different dietary choices and respecting those differences is important.

7.3 Overcoming Common Challenges

While following the Paleo Diet, you might encounter specific challenges. Here are some solutions:

a. Cravings: Cravings for non-Paleo foods are common. Combat them by having Paleo-friendly snacks on hand, such as nuts or sliced vegetables with dip.

b. Social Pressure: Some people may not understand or respect your dietary choices. Politely explain your reasons for following the Paleo Diet, and if they persist, kindly stand your ground.

c. Limited Options: In some situations, Paleo-friendly options may be limited. In such cases, do your best to make the healthiest choices available to you.

d. Time Constraints: Busy schedules can make meal preparation challenging. Plan and prep meals in advance, or find quick and easy Paleo recipes for those hectic days.

e. Travel: Traveling can pose challenges, but with careful planning, you can still stick to your Paleo principles. Research restaurants in advance, bring Paleo-friendly snacks for the journey, and consider renting accommodations with kitchen facilities.

f. Staying Consistent: Consistency is key to success on the Paleo Diet. Develop a routine that works for you, set realistic goals, and stay committed.

while the Paleo Diet has specific guidelines, it's essential to find a balance that suits your individual needs and lifestyle. Flexibility and adaptation are crucial when navigating social situations and overcoming challenges while following the Paleo Diet.

CHAPTER 8

Paleo Diet for Weight Loss

The Paleo Diet is often chosen for its potential to support weight loss while promoting overall health and well-being.

8.1 How the Paleo Diet Supports Weight Loss

The Paleo Diet can support weight loss through several mechanisms:

a. Increased Nutrient Density: Paleo encourages the consumption of nutrient-dense foods like lean meats, vegetables, fruits, and nuts. These foods are filling and provide essential nutrients, helping to curb excessive calorie intake.

b. Reduced Processed Foods: By eliminating processed and refined foods, the Paleo Diet reduces the consumption of empty calories, excessive sugars, and unhealthy fats that can contribute to weight gain.

c. Enhanced Satiety: The diet's emphasis on protein and healthy fats can increase feelings of fullness and satisfaction, reducing the likelihood of overeating.

d. Improved Blood Sugar Control: The Paleo Diet's avoidance of refined sugars and processed carbohydrates can help stabilize blood sugar levels, reducing cravings for sugary snacks.

e. Lower Caloric Intake: Many people naturally consume fewer calories on the Paleo Diet due to the higher satiety of whole foods.

f. Elimination of Problematic Foods: The exclusion of grains and legumes, which can sometimes cause digestive discomfort in some individuals, can lead to a reduction in bloating and water retention.

8.2 Setting Realistic Weight Loss Goals

When embarking on a weight loss journey with the Paleo Diet, it's essential to set realistic and sustainable goals:

a. Be Specific: Define your weight loss goals clearly. For example, specify how much weight you want to lose and by when.

b. Make Goals Measurable: Set measurable goals that can be tracked. This could be a target weight or clothing size.

c. Be Realistic: Ensure that your weight loss goals are achievable and healthy. Rapid, drastic weight loss is often not sustainable and can have adverse health effects.

d. Break Goals into Smaller Steps: Consider breaking your overall goal into smaller, more achievable milestones. Achieving these smaller goals can boost motivation.

e. Focus on Health: While weight loss is a common goal, remember that health and well-being should be the primary focus. Aim for a balanced, nutrient-rich diet that supports your overall health.

f. Seek Support: Consider involving a healthcare professional or registered dietitian in your weight loss journey. They can provide personalized guidance and support.

g. Monitor Progress: Keep a record of your dietary choices, exercise routines, and weight changes. Regular tracking can help you stay accountable and make adjustments when necessary.

8.3 Combining Paleo with Physical Activity

While the Paleo Diet can contribute to weight loss, combining it with regular physical activity can enhance your results and promote overall fitness. Here's how to incorporate exercise into your Paleo weight loss plan:

a. Choose Activities You Enjoy:
Find physical activities that you enjoy, whether it's hiking, cycling, swimming, or dancing. When you enjoy what you're doing, you're more likely to stick with it.

b. Start Slow: If you're new to exercise, start slowly and gradually increase intensity and duration. Overexerting yourself can lead to burnout or injury.

c. Incorporate Strength Training:
Include strength training exercises to build lean muscle mass. Muscle burns more calories at rest than fat, contributing to long-term weight management.

d. Mix Cardio and Strength: A combination of cardiovascular exercises (e.g., jogging, brisk walking) and strength training can be particularly effective for weight loss and overall fitness.

e. Stay Consistent: Consistency is key. Aim for regular, sustainable physical activity rather than sporadic, intense bursts of exercise.

f. Consult a Professional: If you have specific fitness goals or medical considerations, consult with a fitness trainer or physical therapist to create a tailored exercise plan.

weight loss and fitness are individual journeys, and what works for one person may not work for another. It's crucial to listen to your body, make gradual changes, and be patient with your progress. Additionally, consult with a healthcare professional before starting any new diet or exercise program, especially if you have underlying health conditions.

CHAPTER 9

Paleo Diet and Health

The Paleo Diet has gained popularity in part because of its potential health benefits.

9.1 Impact of the Paleo Diet on Health Markers

The Paleo Diet has been associated with several positive changes in health markers:

a. Weight Management: Many people experience weight loss or improved weight management on the Paleo Diet. By emphasizing whole foods and eliminating processed and high-calorie foods, it's easier to control calorie intake.

b. Blood Sugar Control: The Paleo Diet, with its focus on low-glycemic index foods and the avoidance of refined sugars, can help stabilize blood sugar levels. This can be particularly beneficial for individuals with type 2 diabetes or those at risk for the condition.

c. Heart Health: The diet's emphasis on lean meats, fish, nuts, and healthy fats can lead to improvements in heart health. These foods are rich in omega-3 fatty acids, which are known to reduce inflammation and lower the risk of heart disease.

d. Inflammation Reduction: By eliminating processed foods and grains, which can contribute to inflammation, the Paleo Diet may reduce overall inflammation in the body. Chronic inflammation is associated with various chronic diseases.

e. Improved Lipid Profiles: Some studies have shown improvements in lipid profiles, including reduced levels of total cholesterol, LDL cholesterol (the "bad" cholesterol), and triglycerides when following the Paleo Diet. However, these results can vary among individuals.

f. Enhanced Nutrient Intake: The Paleo Diet encourages the consumption of nutrient-dense foods like fruits, vegetables, and lean proteins. This can lead to an increased intake of vitamins, minerals, and antioxidants, which are essential for overall health.

g. Gut Health: The diet's focus on whole foods and the exclusion of processed items can have a positive impact on gut health. A healthy gut microbiome is associated with various aspects of well-being, including digestion and immune function.

h. Satiety and Appetite Control: The Paleo Diet's emphasis on protein, fiber, and healthy fats may enhance feelings of fullness and satiety, which can help control appetite and reduce overeating.

i. Improved Insulin Sensitivity: Some research suggests that the Paleo Diet may improve insulin sensitivity, making it beneficial for individuals with insulin resistance or prediabetes.

It's important to note that while the Paleo Diet has shown promising results in some areas, research is ongoing, and individual responses can vary. The diet may not be suitable for everyone, and it's essential to consult with a healthcare professional before making significant dietary changes, especially if you have underlying health conditions.

The quality of food choices within the Paleo Diet can vary greatly. For optimal health benefits, focus on consuming a variety of nutrient-dense whole foods and maintain a balanced approach to your diet.

9.2 Addressing Concerns and Criticisms

While the Paleo Diet has gained popularity for its potential health benefits, it has also faced criticisms and concerns. Here are some common criticisms and responses to address them:

1. Lack of Whole Grains: Critics argue that the Paleo Diet excludes whole grains, which are a good source of fiber and nutrients.

Response: While it's true that the Paleo Diet excludes grains, it encourages the consumption of other fiber-rich foods such as fruits, vegetables, and nuts. These foods can provide adequate fiber intake. Furthermore, some individuals may find that they don't tolerate grains well, as they can be a source of digestive discomfort for some.

2. Restrictive Nature: Critics claim that the Paleo Diet is too restrictive and difficult to sustain in the long term.

Response: The perceived restrictiveness of the diet can vary among individuals. Some people find it manageable and sustainable, while others may struggle with the limitations. It's essential to adapt the diet to your preferences and lifestyle. While the strictest version of the diet excludes certain food groups, some individuals choose to incorporate limited amounts of dairy or grains, making it less restrictive.

3. Nutrient Gaps: Critics argue that the Paleo Diet may result in nutrient gaps, such as calcium and vitamin D, due to the exclusion of dairy products.

Response: It's possible to obtain sufficient calcium and vitamin D on the Paleo Diet through alternative sources. For example, leafy greens like kale and spinach are rich in calcium, and sunlight exposure contributes to vitamin D synthesis in the body. Additionally, some individuals include small amounts of dairy alternatives like almond milk or fortified coconut milk in their diets.

4. Cost: Some critics claim that the Paleo Diet can be expensive due to the emphasis on high-quality meats and organic produce.

Response: While it's true that organic and grass-fed options can be more expensive, it's possible to follow the Paleo Diet on a budget. Shop for in-season produce, buy frozen fruits and vegetables, and look for sales or discounts on meat. Prioritize spending on foods that align with the diet's principles and adjust your choices based on your budget.

5. Lack of Long-Term Research: Critics argue that there is limited long-term research on the health effects of the Paleo Diet.

Response: Long-term studies on the Paleo Diet are still relatively scarce, but ongoing research is shedding more light on its potential effects. However, it's essential to acknowledge that individual responses to the diet can vary widely. Some people may thrive on it, while others may not experience the same benefits. As with any diet, it's crucial to monitor your health and make adjustments based on your own experiences and needs.

6. Sustainability Concerns: Critics raise concerns about the environmental sustainability of the Paleo Diet due to the increased consumption of animal products.

Response: Sustainable choices within the Paleo Diet are possible. Look for grass-fed, pasture-raised, or sustainably sourced meats and seafood. Additionally, consider incorporating more plant-based proteins, such as nuts, seeds, and legumes, to reduce the environmental impact.

The Paleo Diet has both proponents and critics. It's essential to approach this or any diet with a balanced perspective, considering individual preferences, health goals, and ethical considerations. Consulting with a healthcare professional or registered dietitian can help you make informed decisions about whether the Paleo Diet is suitable for your specific needs and circumstances.

9.3 Consulting a Healthcare Professional

Before making significant dietary changes, especially if you plan to follow a specific diet like the Paleo Diet, it's advisable to consult a healthcare professional or a registered dietitian. Here's why and how to seek their guidance:

1. Personalized Advice: Healthcare professionals can provide personalized advice tailored to your unique health status, medical history, and dietary preferences. They can help you determine if the Paleo Diet is appropriate for you.

2. Health Assessment: A healthcare professional can assess your current health and identify any underlying conditions or risk factors that may impact your dietary choices. This can be crucial in making informed decisions about your diet.

3. Addressing Specific Needs: If you have specific dietary needs or restrictions due to allergies, medical conditions, or cultural preferences, a healthcare professional can help you navigate these challenges within the framework of the Paleo Diet.

4. Monitoring Progress: Healthcare professionals can monitor your progress, including weight loss, changes in health markers, and overall well-being. Regular check-ins can help ensure that the diet is safe and effective for you.

5. Preventing Nutrient Deficiencies: A registered dietitian can help you plan a well-balanced Paleo Diet that meets your nutritional needs and minimizes the risk of nutrient deficiencies. They can provide guidance on supplement use if necessary.

6. Managing Chronic Conditions: If you have chronic health conditions such as diabetes, heart disease, or gastrointestinal disorders, a healthcare professional can help you make dietary choices that support your condition while aligning with the principles of the Paleo Diet.

7. Long-Term Sustainability: Healthcare professionals can assist in developing a dietary plan that is sustainable and aligned with your long-term health goals. They can help you avoid potential pitfalls and challenges associated with the diet.

8. Psychological Support: Changing dietary habits can be emotionally challenging. Healthcare professionals can offer psychological support and strategies for coping with cravings, emotional eating, and the social aspects of diet changes.

How to Consult a Healthcare Professional:

1. **Find a Registered Dietitian:** Look for a registered dietitian (RD) or a registered dietitian nutritionist (RDN) in your area. These professionals are trained to provide evidence-based nutrition advice.

2. **Schedule an Appointment:** Contact the dietitian's office and schedule an appointment. Be prepared to discuss your dietary goals, any medical conditions or allergies, and your current eating habits.

3. **Ask Questions:** During your appointment, don't hesitate to ask questions and seek clarification on any dietary concerns you have. Share your interest in the Paleo Diet and inquire about its suitability for your situation.

4. **Follow the Advice:** Once you've received guidance from a healthcare professional, follow their recommendations and regularly check in for updates or adjustments to your dietary plan.

healthcare professionals can provide valuable insights and support to help you make informed dietary decisions. Their guidance can help ensure that any dietary changes you make, including adopting the Paleo Diet, are safe, effective, and conducive to your long-term health and well-being.

CHAPTER 10

Long-Term Sustainability and Adaptation

Sustainability and adaptability are essential aspects of any dietary approach.

10.1 Making Paleo a Lifestyle, Not a Fad

To ensure that the Paleo Diet remains a sustainable and lasting dietary choice, consider the following strategies:

a. Educate Yourself: Invest time in learning about the principles and science behind the Paleo Diet. Understanding why certain foods are included while others are excluded can reinforce your commitment.

b. Embrace Variety: The Paleo Diet can be diverse and enjoyable. Explore a wide range of fruits, vegetables, meats, and alternative ingredients to keep your meals interesting.

c. Experiment with Recipes: There are countless Paleo-friendly recipes available online and in cookbooks. Experimenting with new recipes can help you discover delicious and creative ways to prepare Paleo meals.

d. Plan Ahead: Meal planning is essential for long-term success. Allocate time each week to plan your meals, create shopping lists, and prepare ingredients in advance to streamline your cooking.

e. Gradual Transition: If you're new to the Paleo Diet, consider making a gradual transition. Start by eliminating processed foods and gradually reduce your intake of grains, legumes, and dairy. This can make the adjustment more manageable.

f. Customize to Your Needs: The Paleo Diet is flexible. Customize it to your dietary preferences and needs. If you find that certain foods or food groups are beneficial for you, consider incorporating them in moderation.

g. Social Support: Share your dietary goals and challenges with friends and family. Engaging in the Paleo Diet as a group or with a supportive network can make it easier to sustain over time.

h. Seek Professional Guidance: Consult with a registered dietitian or healthcare professional to ensure that your dietary choices align with your health goals and individual needs.

i. Listen to Your Body: Pay attention to how your body responds to the Paleo Diet. If you experience any adverse effects or discomfort, be open to making adjustments. It's essential to prioritize your well-being.

j. Practice Mindfulness: Mindful eating involves paying attention to your body's hunger and fullness cues, as well as savoring the flavors of your food. This practice can help you develop a healthier relationship with food and make sustainable dietary choices.

k. Occasional Flexibility: While the Paleo Diet has specific guidelines, occasional flexibility can make it more sustainable. It's okay to enjoy non-Paleo foods on special occasions or when dining out, as long as you return to your chosen dietary approach afterward.

l. Focus on Health: Remember that the primary goal of any diet should be to promote health and well-being. Shift your focus away from weight loss or appearance-related goals and instead prioritize feeling energized and nourished.

Incorporating these strategies into your approach to the Paleo Diet, you can transform it from a short-term fad into a long-term, sustainable lifestyle choice. Sustainability often comes from finding joy and satisfaction in your dietary choices and adapting them to meet your evolving needs and preferences over time.

10.2 Adapting Paleo to Your Changing Needs

As your life and health circumstances change, it's essential to adapt your dietary approach, including the Paleo Diet, to meet your evolving needs. Here's how to adapt the Paleo Diet as your circumstances change:

a. Pregnancy and Nursing: During pregnancy and lactation, your nutritional needs change significantly. Consult with a healthcare provider or registered dietitian to ensure that you're getting adequate nutrients like folate, iron, and calcium. While the Paleo Diet can still be a foundation, it may require adjustments to meet these needs.

b. Childhood and Family: If you have children or family members with different dietary preferences, adapt the Paleo Diet to accommodate everyone's needs. Ensure that children receive sufficient nutrients for growth and development by including nutrient-dense foods like fruits, vegetables, and lean proteins.

c. Athletic Performance: If you're an athlete or engage in regular physical activity, you may require additional carbohydrates for energy. Consider incorporating starchy vegetables like sweet potatoes or occasional grains to support your training and recovery.

d. Age and Life Stages: As you age, your nutritional needs may change. Adapt your diet to support bone health, heart health, and overall well-being. Focus on nutrient-dense foods rich in calcium, vitamin D, and antioxidants.

e. Medical Conditions: If you develop medical conditions such as diabetes, heart disease, or food allergies, work with a healthcare provider or registered dietitian to modify the Paleo Diet to manage your condition effectively.

f. Cultural or Ethical Considerations: If cultural or ethical factors influence your dietary choices, adapt the Paleo Diet to align with your values while still maintaining the core principles of whole foods and avoiding processed items.

g. Seasonal and Environmental Factors: Consider the availability of local and seasonal produce in your area. Embrace fresh, seasonal ingredients to reduce your carbon footprint and support sustainability.

h. Taste Preferences: As your taste preferences evolve, experiment with new recipes and flavor combinations within the Paleo framework to keep your meals enjoyable and satisfying.

10.3 Continuing Your Health Journey

The Paleo Diet can be a starting point for a lifelong health journey. Here are some key considerations for continuing your health journey:

a. Regular Check-Ins: Periodically assess your health, dietary choices, and goals. This can help you make necessary adjustments and ensure that your diet continues to support your well-being.

b. Ongoing Learning: Stay informed about nutrition and health by reading books, articles, and research related to your dietary choices. The field of nutrition is continually evolving, so staying up-to-date is essential.

c. Professional Guidance: Continue to consult with healthcare professionals or registered dietitians for guidance and support as needed. They can provide evidence-based recommendations and help you navigate any health challenges.

d. Mindful Eating: Practice mindful eating to maintain a healthy relationship with food. Be attuned to your body's hunger and fullness cues, and savor the flavors of your meals.

e. Flexibility: Be open to dietary flexibility when necessary, such as during special occasions or when traveling. Adapt to changing circumstances while still prioritizing health.

f. Community and Support: Engage with communities or support groups that share your dietary and health interests. Connecting with others can provide motivation, inspiration, and a sense of belonging.

g. Enjoy the Journey: Remember that your health journey is not just about reaching a destination but enjoying the process. Embrace the joy of cooking, trying new foods, and feeling your best.

Your health journey is a lifelong endeavor, and your dietary choices should evolve with you. Whether you

continue with the Paleo Diet or
explore other approaches, the key is to
prioritize health, well-being, and
sustainability in your dietary
decisions.

www.ingramcontent.com/pod-product-compliance
Lightning Source LLC
Chambersburg PA
CBHW060950260726
48661CB00005B/1820